I0436802

F.A.T. Chronicles

ELIZABETH TISMEER

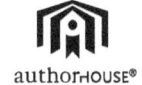

authorHOUSE®

AuthorHouse™
1663 Liberty Drive, Suite 200
Bloomington, IN 47403
www.authorhouse.com
Phone: 1-800-839-8640

First published by AuthorHouse   1/12/2009

ISBN: 978-1-4389-3128-9 (sc)

Printed in the United States of America
Bloomington, Indiana

This book is printed on acid-free paper.

DEDICATION

There is only one woman to dedicate this work to: Dr. Jaclyn Oliva opened the doors of my mind and walked with me through the dark chambers beyond. Once in, our travels together through my past were rocky and precarious. Many times I felt I would not recover from some truths revealed. She never gave up on me, even when I begged to give up on myself. Her professional wisdom and caring gave me strength and courage; her friendship kept me warm. We worked together for eleven years.

Communication: The Aphrodisiac of Intellectuals

and Other Intelligent Beings

CONTENTS

FOREWORD

I am not a PhD. I am an FA—a food addict.
Please read my story. When you get to know me
in the following pages, I hope at some point it will
enlighten you and even make you laugh and cry a
little. Mostly, I hope it brings about some revelation
that will serve to benefit you; my fellow food
addicts, this is for you.

INTRODUCTION

I am a writer; words are my greatest passion! I love to write, and I value greatly the power of the oral and written word. They draw emotions like love, joy, and compassion as well as tears, heartache, and pain. Words are my life. The pen is my sword. When you read further, you will connect this with my personality and characteristics. Writing is a one-person game, an individual sport.

ABOUT ME

As I share my thoughts in this diary, please know I am *fat* today. But the good news is I will not give up on my quest to be the right size. I dream of feeling pleased when I look in the mirror. Currently, when I look in the mirror, the woman looking back is critical of me (her name Julia). Julia has a beautiful face. Her eyes, the size of huge almonds, are deep brown, and there is a blaze behind them that would drop men to their knees (or so she believes ☺). One of the first things she says to me is, "Well, it's about time you came by. I know you've been avoiding me. Well let me tell you, missy, you may not be looking in at me, but I am watching you, and I have not forgotten your promise to buy us new clothes. If I have to go one more year with these frumpy pants, I cannot tell you what I will be capable of ..." She asks me when we are getting our act together, and she hates the clothes I make her wear. She wants tight purple leggings, not baggy sweat pants. She wants slinky, form-fitting, off-the-shoulder tops, not oversized T-shirts made specifically for hiding the rolls underneath. She is shameful, really. Would you believe she wants to display her ample cleavage in public? What a diva! I must say, though, she does have lovely breasts and a nice figure when she is the right size. I have asked her to keep her (baggy) pants on, and she will get her wishes. But she remains impatient.

My last words to her for today are, "*Patience is its own reward, Julia.*"

We have lots of work to do …

I could say here how much I weigh, but it has no significance to anyone but me. I can tell you how many pounds or inches I want to lose, but again, no significance. I want to right-size. Right-sizing is very subjective. I have a vision of the ideal body for me. That will vary with every human being, so for the purpose of this writing I say to one and all, you set up your objectives for your right size. No one can have a vote except if you give them a vote. It is our choice; as for me, mine is the only vote that matters. What is *fat* to others is *phat* to me, baby! I have empowered myself on this subject, and that's all I want to say about it.

Over the years I, like others, have tried every way possible to right-size—yes, all the traditional mainstream fad diets, and some not-so-mainstream ones like contraband diet pills. This was totally

Loserville. You know the payback for this behavior.

I am a drug addict! My drug of choice is *food*.
Like any worthy drug addict, I know how to get
a hold of my stash. For example, the vending
machine at work (a landmine) holds Cheetos (A3),
Honey buns (D1), and Snickers (F5). But my diary
is about losing the food addiction and gaining self-
esteem.

All in all, it's in the brain. Every diet plan works
when you work it. Discipline is the key, but also
key is dedication to yourself—loving yourself more
than you love the drug. I don't want my diary to be
about what I ate today or whether I was "good" or
not. It is much more than that.

I have decided as a first step to confront my fears:

- Being right-sized will make me promiscuous.
- Being right-sized will invite unwelcome attention.
- Being right-sized will make me a target of sexual predators.
- Being right-sized will distract me from my goals.
- Being right-sized could make me vain.
- Being right-sized will make me vulnerable.

Enough Already!

Elizabeth, leave your fears on this page. They are no longer valid.

Pledges

- I pledge that I will always protect myself.
- I pledge that I will maintain a healthy lifestyle.

- I pledge to stay focused on my goals.

- I pledge to love myself and embrace my right-sized body without fears.

- I pledge to let go of the baggage from my past.

- I pledge to love myself first.

- I pledge to surround myself with good and trustworthy friends.

Mind Games: "Eat to Live"

Every morning, I will write down my meal plan and stick with it.

- I will take out a pair of jeans that I love but don't currently fit in. I will try them on once a week on the same day and at the same time.

- I will put away the scale. The only thing that matters to me is *inches*.

- Whenever the cravings return, I will drink a large glass of water instead.

- I will give myself permission to have a low-fat treat at lunch from time to time.

- I will distract myself with other activities.

- I will exercise. I hate to exercise, but I know I must.

Failure Only Exists When You Fail to Get Up After Being Knocked Down

CHAPTER ONE

Many have walked this path before, but these footprints belong to me.

All my life I have been an addict. My drugs of choice have ranged from alcohol to tobacco to food (the other "f" word). This diary is about my food addiction and about the battles fought and lost. But more than that, it is about winning the war. I decided to record my fight, to give myself some leverage by holding myself accountable for my decisions, and to hear what actually goes on in my mind as I either give in to or resist the allure of the foods I crave.

I'm a food addict, and I have been struggling like you cannot believe—or maybe some of you can—with drug addiction. Food is a drug; it's my drug of choice, and it is defeating me almost every day. I am creating this diary because I don't want this addiction. I want to win the war. Way, way, way too many battles have been lost at this point in time. I'm at the end of my ability to do this quietly. I need to speak out now. I'm hoping this diary will serve as a weapon against this food addiction. I'm hoping that by voicing it, by giving it visibility, it will lose some of its power over me. I am totally at my wits' end. I don't want to admit this, but I know that I am. I've always had an addictive personality; it's in my genes. I will say here that I have conquered other addictions. I used to smoke.

Thinking back about the smoking addiction,

I find it interesting that after smoking from age fourteen to approximately age twenty-eight, I quit smoking because my new boyfriend was a nonsmoker and he asked me to quit—so I did. I recall that I did not have withdrawal issues, nor did I struggle with cravings. I simply decided that I liked the boyfriend more than I liked cigarettes. There was no trauma or denial in the interim.

Long story short, I married the boyfriend. We divorced after fourteen years of marriage. However, I have never given cigarettes a second thought. I used to drink heavily....

Wouldn't it go hand in hand? I started drinking at the same time that I had my first cigarette. My father was an alcoholic. Almost every adult around me when I was growing up drank heavily, except my mom. It was a way of life. Naturally, I gravitated toward booze as soon as I could. I did not stop until nine years ago. I am also an alcoholic. I am an alcoholic who is dry. Now, this diary is not about alcoholism. But because it is about addictions, I must admit to all my addictions. I fell deeply into the abyss that is alcoholism. I spent many of my early years hating myself because alcohol brought out the whore in me. It brought out the daring, no-holds-barred, reckless, self-destructive, self-loathing woman in me. How I hated myself when I sobered up. It was so bad at one point that I can say I am very lucky today I did not kill someone when I drank and got behind the wheel. Some mornings, I could not recall how I got home. I was so out of control. Sadly, during this period, the shame I felt was so great that I could not ask for help in the traditional ways like Alcoholics Anonymous (AA). Back then I was pretty good at hiding my alcoholism because I was a binge drinker. In short, there was no one to help me.

After I married, by my own sheer will, I began
to control the drinking binges. I had a new
husband and a step-son in my life. But alcohol was
still controlling me during my marriage and carried
on after I was divorced. Then one day in January,
2000, I finally reached out to the heavens and
demanded help. I sat in my kitchen one afternoon
and shook my fist toward the sky as I swore at God.
I was in such despair. I told Him that I wanted to
die, and if He was really out there, he had to come
now, or I would kill myself. That afternoon, two
strangers came to my rescue. This is a story for
another time, but suffice it to say, I have not had
another drink since …

When I first decided to record my thoughts
about my food addiction, I knew I had to be
brutally honest with myself. I needed to pull
out every skeleton in the closet, every shameful
behavior related to food, and I needed to be

courageous and bold. Otherwise what is the point? There is no sugar coating here. I am going to be raw about this. The other day I bought a voice recorder, and I knew I would not hold anything back. All the warts and blemishes that I am comprised of will be revealed.

Growing Up

Before I begin, however, I believe it is important to share that I had a very "difficult" childhood. I am not making excuses, but growing up was a matter of survival. I suffered greatly along with my siblings. I am the youngest of four children. My brothers and sister suffered their own way and have their own memories, but there was a commonality among our individual and unique experiences. I won't tell their stories because they are not for me to tell; I will only tell you mine.

As a little girl, I was molested by several male

adult family members. In a twisted sort of way, I almost believe I was lucky because the abuse was not pervasive as in other children's experiences I have heard of but it did have a profound effect on me none the less. The shame that I feel never goes away. Unfortunately, as with many of my sisters in the world, when I finally told my mother, she did not believe me. I can only guess it was simply easier not to believe so that she would not have to deal with it or have feelings about it. I did not have the traditional mother and father figures who took their parental obligations seriously. They simply did not know how. They had their own weaknesses and overall dysfunctions to deal with. Truth be told, they had no business having children. My mother was forced to leave me with extended family members while she went to work. She left me in so many different places that I constantly worried that she would forget where she dropped me off. Quite often I was left for days and weeks before she returned to take me home again. No matter, it was always an eternity for me. I yearned relentlessly for my mother. I have abandonment issues, anxiety, and depression as a result of those experiences. Can anyone blame me for soothing myself with food? Can anyone blame me for cloaking myself with layers of fat as protection against adult predators? I ask myself these questions in order to forgive me for what may be perceived as taking the easy way out. Just smoke, just drink, just eat, eat, eat.

Over the years, I have gained and lost and gained and lost weight. The most severe time was during the mid-eighties. After I got married, I ballooned up to 232 pounds on a 4 foot 11 inch frame. It was grueling to exist in this obesity. My husband used me to get laughs from friends and family. I soothed myself with my arsenal of drugs. After I divorced him, I lost 87 pounds, and he had to find new fodder for his standup act …

Since then, I have regained some of the pounds back. This is where I am today. In the past two and half years, I have been losing more battles than I have been winning. That is why I have decided to go into therapy with myself. I am my therapist and my patient. Why, you ask?

I want to do this on my own this time. I was in therapy throughout most of my marriage; approximately eleven years. Believe me, I have great faith in the therapeutic process, and I am incorporating everything I learned in therapy into this project. (Note: In therapy, I was introduced to my inner family. I met Mom, Dad, and myself as a small child living in poverty. I call her Little One, she is three years old.) I cannot give anyone advice or suggest what any one individual should do in their personal crisis involving food; I can only share my thoughts, ideas, and background.

Chapter Two

Addictions

What are some of the details and facets of my addiction? What does my food addiction consist of? I am one who binges. I am known to run into the grocery store, dash straight to the bakery section, and grab a dozen pastries or a lemon meringue pie, then sit in the car and devour my stash. I will sit in the car with powdered sugar coating my lips, and I have a pretty good rush going. It is euphoric! It's like lounging on a cloud of cotton candy. I love sweets, pastries, pies, sweet rolls, donuts, muffins, cakes, ice cream, and chocolate. I also love all kinds of food. I love Mexican, Italian, Chinese, Japanese, Thai, Indonesian, Indian, and Greek. But when I am on a binge, I mostly go after bakery goods. You see, it's easy to hide in the car and demolish a beautiful German chocolate cake or inhale a few lovely glazed donuts before heading home. Drive-thru restaurants are also pretty handy for hiding in the car with bags of tacos or cheeseburgers and fries. Most of the time, however, I go for sugar. Either way, food addicts find a way to satisfy the cravings. Whether I am binging in the car or at home, nothing lasts for very long. In fact, I keep very little food at home because what I bring home is devoured pretty quickly. If you open my refrigerator, it is pretty barren. I usually have a jar of mayonnaise, pickles, milk, maybe some bagels and cream cheese. My pantry contains cereal, oatmeal, Crystal Light, and other generic dry goods—nothing I would rip into during a craze. I kid myself by never keeping the good drugs at home. Besides, like I said, they wouldn't last for long! For me, part of the high is standing in front of the bakery shelves, salivating over rows and rows of delicious pastries, and knowing that I will relish the chosen few in the very next moments.

The Downside

Unfortunately, the downside of my behavior inevitably circles around, and payback begins. Sometimes my stomach hurts, and I feel nauseated. Then the negative self-talk begins. A member of my inner family appears. The Mother. She chastises me for giving in to the Little One. She berates me and scolds with a wagging finger and angry accusing eyes. She calls me a failure and a loser over and over again.

I start to feel defeated and weak. The addiction beat me again. Simply speaking, if I am in a battle and I surrender to the enemy, then I have been defeated. The Mother is right. Her tirade continues:

"Where's your discipline? Why are you such a wimp? You are useless. You are a worm. You deserve to be a fat pig; you have no spine or backbone. I am ashamed of you, and you should be ashamed of yourself! Go look at your pitiful self in the mirror. Do you like what you see? You are disgusting." The price I pay for my addiction is *big*.

Act One, Scene Two: A Softer Voice, A Forgiving Voice

OK. Don't be so hard on yourself, Elizabeth. Next time, you will be stronger. Next time you will not find the bakery. Next time you will love yourself more than you love the sugar ...

But it's all a façade. I make these declarations while I still have the drug in my body. The voracious worm is satiated for the moment. The Little One has settled down. She feels victorious. Who am I kidding? It's all a fake. I'm a fake. I am languishing in the drug.

Next time ...

My inner family is an obstacle that still drives my unconscious need to stay fat. They have tremendous power over me. The most powerful of all is the Little One who resides in a special place in my heart and still has vivid memories of our childhood. She recalls how vulnerable we were. She recalls being afraid of the dark. *They came in the dark ...* She worries that we will call attention to ourselves and will be exposed like we were before. Simply, she is afraid of being right-sized and being considered pretty and appealing to men. She is the one who is leading the charge when I binge on pastries. I must write her a letter to help her believe and trust in me.

It Is Safe To Be Thin...

Dear Little One:

I want to tell you that I am working on a plan to

lose weight. I want your help, and I want to reassure you that it is safe to be thin. We must stop being afraid to be thin. We are together now. One of us is a grown-up. I am here to take care of both of us. Please trust me when I tell you that from here forward you will never be hurt again. I will protect you from anyone who tries to hurt you. Please understand that your health is at stake. We have to be a healthy weight so we can be beautiful inside and out.

All of the monsters have died, my love. They don't exist anymore. You can sleep sweetly without fear. You can play without looking over your shoulder. You don't have to lock yourself in the bathroom and pray for Mom to come home. I am your mom now. You don't have to be afraid. I am your protector! I love you, my sweet darling.

Elizabeth

Chapter Three

Facing the Demons

Now that I have isolated and identified the demons in my life, I can now address them and face them head on. From today forward I am recording my thoughts and actions. My hope is to discover the patterns and habits I have acquired that drive my food addiction.

Triggers

- ❖ Stress triggers binges.
- ❖ Loneliness and aloneness triggers binges.
- ❖ Boredom triggers binges.

❖ Anxiety triggers binges.

❖ Depression triggers binges.

❖ Conflicts trigger binges.

Only the present matters. In AA, they speak of taking it one day at a time. How will I incorporate that into my personal challenge to lose weight?

Just as a side note, I should say that I have tried Weight Watchers in the recent past. This is an excellent program, but I dropped out after only a few meetings. I was not comfortable in the group setting.

You see, I am a loner. I am an isolationist to a great degree. Not surprising, I know. I am somewhat of a contradiction because I love people but I also love the time I spend alone surrounded by books, computer, TV, music, and food. When I am alone, in the car or at home, I don't have to explain my eating habits. I don't have to apologize when I binge. I believe many addicts are loners for the same reasons.

My point is, I am hoping with all of my heart that others will become aware of my diary and that it will help other food addicts. I love to help and give of myself. I want it to become a tool—a sword, if you will—to help others with their battle, whatever their battle is …

Food is unlike other addictions because we must consume food to live. It's not like cigarettes or alcohol; we cannot disown it completely. I liken it to being locked in a room with a rattlesnake. We have to live with it in the room—it serves a purpose. Food addicts will have a love-hate relationship with the snake. We love the snake when it guards the room from predators, but we hate it too because we know that it can strike at us anytime. We must always protect ourselves from snakebites. To lose the snake is to die.

As a food addict, I must create an environment that is safe and comforting. It must be structured and planned. I must know what I am going to consume in advance, and I must plan meals accordingly. This is a challenge for a person who has an abstract, random personality. I will call my good food list "Edible Edibles." Edibles that are mouth-watering delights, that satisfy hunger but also satisfy the palate and, most important, the brain. In addition, from here on out, I will create a "Poison Dart" list. This list will consist of all the foods that are no longer allowed in my body while I am working on my program.

Once done, I have to identify how I will manage my food intake. As we all know, it isn't just about the right foods; it is also very important to control intake. It's known as portion control. This will be big for me because I gorge myself—remember the lemon meringue pie? *I want it all right now.* That said, how do I choose the right portions and stick to it?

I am an abstract and random personality. I live in grays; the black and white in my life consist of two narrow lines on the left and right of my world. While I believe there is a need for structure in life, I have to stretch to maintain it. However, part of my success will be to sign a contract with myself. I will incorporate balance and structure into my plan (details to follow).

I have to figure it out and do my best—there is no other option.

The things I have figured out right at the beginning of my journey are that pounds don't matter from this point forward. Scales don't matter.

The only thing that matters is how I look and feel. I will measure success by the size clothes I wear. The scale is another enemy, another critic, and I don't need anymore critics beside the one in my brain, thank you very much.

Note: Words give visibility to all of that which we are. This is about me right now, so I just need to give a wide perspective, a big picture of myself, not just as a food addict but as a human being. In short, as an adult I have become kind and good and decent. *I am a "worker bee". When my mother left me places, she would always say these parting words: "Don't just sit around; make yourself useful until I come back for you...". My mother's commands are tatoo'd on my brain so I inevitably incorporated this mentality in all aspects of my adult life; and they served me well in my personal life, and in the workplace, over the years.* Laughter is like oxygen to me. I have compassion and understanding of the human heart. I am intelligent in the area of communication, and I am loyal to those who are loyal to me. I love the movies (and buttered popcorn), I love to read, and my heart soars when I write.

CHAPTER FOUR

Society and Fat People

Society has labeled fat people as insignificant. Society equates fat with stupid because we are unable to control our weight—it makes us *less than*. We are often dismissed and discounted. Well to that I say …

Another of my dreams and aspirations is to become a motivational speaker! And I have known successes not only in the corporate arena but in having conquered smoking and alcohol addictions. I can't explain how I conquered these demons, but I can say I am tenacious and stubborn; some just call me bullheaded. So take that, society!

In all honesty I should also state that there have been (many) times when I have hesitated due to lack of confidence in my appearance. For instance, I won't ask a question or make a comment in a meeting because I don't want eyes upon me. I do feel intimidated by how I perceive that society, my peers, or superiors may view me.

In order to feel credible, I must start by motivating myself. I must win this war I am waging on food. I must create a mental picture of me at my right-size. Then I must become that person.

For now, I can only encourage myself to speak out and be heard no matter how much I weigh at a given time. I know, easier said than done, but doable nonetheless.

Another aspect of society and fat people is how men treat fat women. Generally speaking, the majority of men will immediately dismiss a heavy-set woman outright. He feels ashamed to be with a fat woman. For men, women are a badge of honor. They would prefer to be with a woman who is not particularly pretty as long as she is thin or has a "great body." How often have you heard someone say, "She has such a pretty face, but she is fat, so forget it"?

On the other hand, it is a lot easier for a fat man to find love than it is for a fat woman. Women are very tolerant of fat or "out of shape" men. We forgive easily if a man is no longer in shape. It doesn't matter in most cases. We don't measure our men with the same ruler, and they don't have to abide by the same rules of attraction. Sad but true.

CHAPTER FIVE

Identify the Landmines

I've talked about a lot of things; I have a lot to say. I think that part of the success of my program that I am developing here is I must identify or label other factors that hinder me and fuel the food addictions.

What about the landmines that surround me? I speak of being in a war with food and the many battles I am in, so what about the battlefields? I want to identify the battlefields before I go further. The reason is I must avoid those battlefields at all costs.

The first one that comes to mind is the bakery inside my favorite supermarket. The bakery is a magnet for me. I struggle every moment I spend in the store. I have to find detours that will keep me away from going near the bakery while I shop for other staples. If the supermarket is a battlefield, I consider the bakery one of the landmines on the battlefield.

Next, I must label two donut shops that bake the best pastries. I find freshly baked goods there. I don't even leave the parking lot. I sit in the car and take one bite out of each different pastry until I have lovingly savored all of them. Then I take the second bite, and so it goes. On a good day, so to speak, I have become sick to my stomach, and I get out of the car and throw away the half-eaten portions instead of taking them home for the next round …

Note: One other significant change for me will be when I can think of pastries not as poison but a special treat that I give myself now and then. Of course, I am far and away from this, but I want to keep it in mind and strive to remove all the negativity I feel around certain foods. I strive to have a healthy relationship with my body and with all foods. I want to consider food as nourishment and fuel. I want to focus on food as it gives me energy and strength. I will place this in my Goals List.

CHAPTER SIX

At My Wits' End

I need to stop for a moment to explain in more detail the reasons why I decided to create a diary about my food addiction. I mentioned earlier that I am at my wits' end. I am.

In the past three days I have been on an uncontrollable binge. When it was finally over, I not only felt sick in my stomach, I realized how severe my addiction had become. Something just clicked in my brain. Surely I have been on a million binges, but this time I was scared coming out of this latest spiral downward. I tell you, if it wasn't nailed down, it went into my mouth. I felt devastated and helpless and so miserable.

I sat at home alone just thinking about what to do. I cannot continue this pattern. But what am I to do?

I started thinking about the programs I see advertised on TV but quickly realized I would not stick with them. I would just be wasting my money. I knew that I had to do figure out a plan that is suitable to my personality and my type of addiction.

The solution that came was this diary. I would record all my behaviors and thoughts and binges. I would use these recordings in order to analyze what triggers the binges. What emotions do I feel when decide to gorge myself? What is going on internally and externally? I already knew that I rarely waited to be physically hungry to give myself permission to eat. I am an emotional eater and binger. In fact, I don't believe I recall what physical hunger is really like anymore.

At this time I am saying enough is enough. I cannot live another day without trying to do something to help myself. I don't have a magic potion, but I desperately want to love myself, and I want my inner family to love me unconditionally. I want their help! I need their help …

CHAPTER SEVEN

Where to Start

❖ I will start by choosing a new super market.

❖ I will always have a food list—no random shopping.

❖ I will stop driving near the two favorite donut shops.

❖ I will forbid myself from eating *anything* in the car.

❖ I will shop for healthy finger foods and keep them near at all times.

❖ I will keep myself busy so that I am not thinking about food.

- ❖ I will always bring my lunch to work.
- ❖ I will drink water instead of
  ___.*fill in the blank*
- ❖ I will *exercise.*

I hate exercising, but I do have a treadmill and an elliptical. There are no excuses for not exercising. But I know I will have to slowly incorporate exercise because I don't want to sabotage myself by piling on too much at once. I know how I am, and I must start out by being reasonable about what I need to do. One step at time, one day at a time—like they say at AA.

Geez, the juices are flowing. I am thinking about this new focus. It's really hard when you are thinking about a nutritional program. (I don't like to use the word diet because I think of it as another four-letter word, not to mention it has the word "die" in it.) This is going to require planning. I am worth it. I want eating to become a natural flow in my day, like inhaling and exhaling. I want to eat to sustain my life.

Up to now my life consists of bakeries, fast foods, and vending machines. Fortunately I can eliminate these from my life while I incorporate healthy foods to replace them.

The other important key to my success is to satisfy the palate because that is the only way to keep the brain happy. Since my problem is not about hunger, I must feel that my emotions and my brain are satisfied with my food intake. This is the only way to ensure that I can maintain this conversion in my lifestyle.

I should also note here that I don't cook. I have never been interested in cooking, and I have no desire to incorporate cooking into my new program. The way I look at it, I have been a working woman for almost my entire life. I believe that if I am out breaking a sweat all day long, I deserve to be served a meal at the end of the day. I will have to eat well at home or in restaurants by making right choices and managing portions.

I am not a planner per se. As I have mentioned, I have what is called an abstract random personality, with some concrete and sequential lines drawn in. Note: I have taken many personality profile tests that are structured to identify our four main personality traits. I have two dominant personality traits known as *Abstract and Random*. That is, I tend to live in the gray areas versus the black and white. The two least dominant of my personality traits are, *concrete and sequential.* That said, I live most comfortably in the gray areas. I must call upon the concrete part of my personality in order to plan meals, and the sequential part to help with timing meals. These behaviors do not come naturally for me. Concrete, sequential requires thought and deliberateness. Conversely, living in the "gray areas" is home-so to speak. There resides my creative heart. This is the place where I write. It feels safe and comfortable. Here I can roam anywhere my mind takes me. I can randomly change directions as I choose. I am like a child playing in a toy store with free reign to play as my child's heart desires!

I am a person of such opposite extremes. I say one thing and I live another. At any rate, I am recording everything. I am not just a woman on a weight loss program. I am a woman on a mission to figure myself out better. I am searching for a way to deal with food issues. I cannot make any miraculous improvements. I am in a process.

I don't have to account to anyone except myself. If I had to report my meals to someone, I believe

I would feel defensive, and that is a defeatist emotion.

I have just stopped for gas. It seems every single gas station has a food mart or convenience store. There is simply no getting away from junk food! Lucky for me, I have already had a meal, and I am satisfied right now. The point here is there are drugs everywhere. I can't even stop for gas without being assaulted by the drug and its peddlers. Man alive! Would a regular person even notice or care?

On this note, I just recalled another incident surrounding the drugs … The other day, when I decided to buy the voice recorder, I was standing in line at Best Buy to pay, and right in front of the long row of cashier counters, there are stacks and rows of chips, candies, and soda. It is now 7 p.m. I have not eaten since about 3 p.m. I am eying a bag of Cheetos. I literally start to salivate. This is a struggle! Please, please hurry; let me pay so I can get out of here! The drugs are everywhere; that's my point.

CHAPTER EIGHT

Useful Tools

One of the tools I use to help get past the cravings is a self-talk that I give myself. It goes like this: "Little One, look, just be strong today! If you still want that particular drug tomorrow, you can have it. Honest, just walk away from it today. If you still want it by tomorrow morning, you have permission to eat it." The good thing about this strategy is it works, because by morning, I don't want it anymore; the craving has passed. Sometimes nothing I say to myself works; sometimes I just crash and burn. That's when she says, "Elizabeth, shut up and get out of my way!" The consequences don't matter. I want what I want, when I want it. I will deal with the guilt afterward. The drug is powerful and selfish. I know today that the binging comes from not having enough to eat when I was growing up. I learned pretty quickly that if I did not devour every morsel in front of me, there may not be any later. So …

Luckily, I have taken care of myself financially since I was seventeen years old. I have worked hard and have always had the comforts of life since then. Still, old habits and old memories die hard. I realize I must put that excuse away. I must retire that memory and keep in mind that there will always be plenty tomorrow, and the next day, and the next day.

This Diary, My Best Effort

Still, I know for a fact that the best weapon

for me is to talk this through. Keep the words flowing. Words, for me, have power. I am so tired of keeping the dirty little secrets that really are not so dirty—they are just human. Truly, the only secret to my success is to rationalize, use common sense, and love myself and my inner family. We can win! My Little One has to learn that we have enough to eat. She doesn't have to gorge herself for fear there will be none later. She doesn't have to worry about being cute. She has a protector now. I must not dismiss her presence in my life. I must not dismiss her feelings and her fears; they are real, and they must be acknowledged and worked through.

CHAPTER NINE

Day to Day

I am shopping right now, and I am walking through racks of summer attire. There are lots of shorts and sleeveless T-shirts. I will not buy anything today. This is just another motivator to stay in my program. Stay high for life. I am looking in the size that I used to wear. You know, when I am at my right-size, I look pretty appealing. I am longing now to wear this size again. Food is the furthest from my mind at this moment. There is so much excitement just in shopping when a woman is proud of her body. It doesn't matter what her body looks like; it only matters that she feels good in it. Frankly, my right-size may seem fat to someone else. But for me, I feel grand. None of that matters. We have the *right to choose our right-size*.

I used to fool myself to provide an excuse to buy clothes when I am into the bigger sizes. I say, "Elizabeth, buy your right-size, and it will motivate you to get into them." That tactic has never worked. They stay stuck in the closet with the tags on them. Today, if I buy anything at all, it would only be shoes or purses. Shoes and purses are never critical. They slide on your feet or on your arm. Size doesn't matter to shoes and purses.

OK, I am about to get on the battlefield (supermarket). It is time to put on the armor (discipline) and load my weapons (resistance and focus). I have a list with me. I can easily navigate because I know exactly which aisles I will go to. I can pick up the items on my list and make my exit. This is a great strategy. I must be sure to have a list with me before stepping onto this battlefield. The battle should be brief, and I should emerge victorious. *Always have a list.*

I should point out here that I do have one safety zone. My home! Ironically, it is the same place where I am known to binge. It is simple to explain, really. As a given, I rarely have the foods I love and crave in my house. One reason is they get devoured pretty quickly after they arrive. Also, I don't cook, so I don't have leftovers in the fridge. Ninety percent of the time, I must get in the car and locate my drug dealer. Once I do that, I ingest right in my car! The drug rarely makes it home.

From now on, I will fight the desire to get in the car and find the drug dealer. Instead I will begin to keep healthy foods in the house and carefully keep my meal plan for the day.

One of the things I learned at Weight Watchers is the point system. This is the best because you can eat the foods that you enjoy and lose weight as long as you control the portions. It is so easy with the point system. Satisfying the brain is most important. Let's face it, folks: if your brain is not satisfied, you are going to continue searching for something to put in your mouth. It has nothing to do with hunger or need. The brain does not rest until it is satiated.

Because I am aware that I am an emotional eater, I have used food to soothe myself. I get that rush and that lovin' feelin' that the Righteous Brothers sang about back in the '60s. I want to learn to use food as a form of nourishment not for emotional comfort. I know I can do this; it will take time and lots of mental practice. Acknowledgment and visibility is part of the road to success. This diary acknowledges and brings forth visibility in its pages, in black and white.

Chapter Ten

Breaking It Down

I realize in all of this that I am only as good as the next thirty seconds, the next meal. I want to keep my focus- only on each day. I don't want to worry about tomorrow or next month. The only thing that matters in life (and right-size programs) is what I do *today*. Successes come in snippets, in segments of time—not days and weeks and months, but moment by moment.

Being aware, alert, and most of all prepared is also important.

Speaking of Awareness, some other bad habits to be aware of and discard are saying to myself that the day is a failure when I blow it, and I might as well forget about my plan and eat whatever I want. Not good. I must say "That was one moment, but the rest of the day still matters." I must get back on plan. Success comes in the moment, in the present. Don't look back; just keep looking forward.

Did I Say Patience Is Its Own Reward?

All of my life I have been a "now" person. As a child, I believed I had to eat everything in my sight because there may not be any food later. Poverty instills an anxiety in the poor. They are on a constant search for sustenance. They are surviving moment by moment. Poverty has manifested in me a few idiosyncrasies that I will share with you:

- I eat very fast.

- I bite off more than I can chew.

- I don't chew properly.

- I always overload my plate.

- I forget to drink water during meals.

- I constantly eat passed feeling full.

- I clean my plate.

- I am a glutton.

I Am Learning To:

- Slow down.

- Chew, chew, chew.

- Pick up small portions on my fork.

- Use salad plates, not large dinner plates.

- Drink one 8 oz. glass of water before each meal.

- Drink water during my meal.

- Put down my fork between bites.

- Savor the food in my mouth.

- Remove all distraction and enjoy each morsel.

- Eat like a lady, like a Southern belle.

- Have a low-fat dessert on Saturdays, if I wish.

- *Remember that there will be more food at the next meal time.*

Speaking of the Now ...

I want to stay in the moment with my program. Although I can plan for the day, I don't want to think too far ahead at any given time. I will be aware and prepared for morning mealtime and not think about snack time or lunch. Getting through the next thirty minutes will be fine for me. I believe that will work best. For the next thirty minutes I am going to be successful in my program. Later, as I become accustomed to it, I can stretch to an hour at a time and so on … I believe this is the best way to manage it. What matters is good nutrition, portion control, and drinking water. I want a balanced routine that contains lots of variety and satisfies the stomach and the brain.

CHAPTER ELEVEN

Deprivation

A lot of us want to punish ourselves when we are fat. We want to punish ourselves for not having control to maintain our right-size. We begin to subtly and not so subtly deprive ourselves of so-called privileges that we enjoy. If you are like me, you are already struggling to deprive yourself of the foods that you love but make you fat. That's plenty to manage. I want to declare now that I will stop doing that. I deserve to get manicures and pedicures. I deserve to shop if I feel like shopping; it doesn't matter if I don't buy. Shopping is fun. I want to continue to treat myself while I am in my program and not say, "After I lose the weight, I will …"

Deprivation No More!

From now on I will focus on successes I have had and treat myself for my successes in other areas of my life, no matter how big or small. Besides, I believe treating myself will give me encouragement to continue right-sizing! It's all in the brain, gals and guys. If you are a person who is juggling work with parenting and all that entails, you are a success. If you get your kids off to school on time and arrive at work on time, you are a success. If you get grocery shopping done and get dinner on the table that evening, you are a success. Shall I stop now, or do I need to add, laundry, housekeeping, yard work, homework, bath time, and bedtime stories, not to mention Fido and Garfield?

While we are on the subject, I have to say that

the one thing that I have always seen to is being as presentable as possible regardless of my size. I take great care to wear the right makeup, have my hair styled, and dress in a manner that still accentuates the positive. Since I have always been a working woman, I feel I should show up to the office in a manner that is appropriate for the business environment. I never wanted to lower the bar just because I am fat. I want to look my best regardless of what my best is in a given time. The way I see it, people have to engage with me and interact with me all day. They may already be distracted by my body size. I don't want them to be distracted by my overall appearance, too.

CHAPTER TWELVE

Lapses

I have made a declaration not to allow a lapse [from my program] to give me permission to blow off the whole day. Of course, if you're like me, that is not easy. But I can do it if I talk the Little One into getting back on the right track right away. That is going to mean I must continue to talk to the Little One and tell her that I have given in to her this time but that this behavior must stop.

The Little One is incredibly stubborn and tenacious. She had to be strong and resourceful in order to find ways to take care of herself when the Mother was absent. She depended only on herself on many days. I am so grateful to her for not giving in or giving up. That said, she cannot let go of her memories. She still reacts to life from a basis of her childhood. She trusts but she doesn't trust. She believes grown-ups are bad. Men cannot be trusted. And she eats every chance that she can, because later ...

I have to keep talking to her. She is at the core of my success. I know that if I can bring her around and get her to believe how sincere I am and how much I love her, she will begin to feel safe. That is when she will start to peel away the fears and let go of her pain. I long for the day when she will place her faith in me and allow me to make all the decisions for us.

I have already shared the reasons why she still

doesn't trust me. I have made plenty of wrong choices in my adult life. I don't believe this diary is the forum for going into even more detail surrounding my adult life, so I will save that for another diary. In the meantime, I will strive to show her that I have learned my lessons, and she doesn't have to worry anymore.

Chapter Fourteen

What's Love Got to Do with It

I will say, however, that I do want to be loved someday! Sure, I would love it if a man could love me as I am today. But in my experience, this is not realistic. So to be loved means I must be right-sized and be visually appealing to men. In my lifetime, [Julia] and I have received attention from men, but for all the wrong reasons. It was not about love at all, and unfortunately I did not see the light until after I was hurt deeply.

In the meantime, I work. I stay busy with my

personal interests and a handful of friends that I love very much. And I enjoy my private time. But I must admit it isn't always what I want … In life there is a cost for everything. The price we pay for being alone is loneliness. I try not to let this beast creep in, but sometimes he does, and he often overstays his welcome.

I have no idea today if I will find that life partner, but I will keep hoping because I believe in love and companionship. I want to touch a man's life in the most positive way. I want to make him laugh and feel excited when he hears my voice on the phone or hears my car in the driveway. I want him to feel a rush throughout his body when he is in the next room and hears me moving about. I want my heart to beat one hundred times its normal speed when he holds me and makes passionate love to me. I want us to speak to each other with our eyes, and I want our hearts to still be entwined when we are apart. The harmony of two hearts beating in love for each other—that's what love has to do with it.

CHAPTER FIFTEEN

The Father

The Father does not play as big a role as the Little One and the Mother do in my inner family. Rather, he sits quietly, legs crossed, a guitar on his lap. Until now, I could not allow him into my heart. I have a powerful sense of him that consists of deep pain and sadness blended together. These emotions stand between us like a brick wall. Abandonement lies at his feet where my heart is; loss and neglect linger nearby … I am too cowardly to ask him to pick me up and hold me. If I give him entrance into my heart, he will surely break it.

The sober Father was very kind, very giving and very, very charming. He was also very talented. He loved music. He taught himself how to play guitar. His only legacy was in the music. As such, he not only entertained with his charm, but that guitar bedazzled everyone near. He also had a showman personality; he was always on stage. Everyone loved being around him, when he was sober.

When he drank he was evil and violent. He went after the Mother with such hatred and vengeance. He beat her often. All I could do was cry.

The Father did not raise me. He was either drunk at home or away on a drunken binge. He also spent lots of his time in the county jail. In fact, he was taking up residence in the county jail when I was born. We did not lay eyes on each other until I was over a year old. He was finally expelled from the family when I was fifteen. My oldest brother drove him to the bus station and told him he should never return. Thereafter, I only saw him for a few hours in between the decades that followed. He died in 2003. I attended his funeral because it was the right thing to do.

The Mother

I have written about the Mother that resides inside me. The Mother that I grew up with must be commended now. She did not discard us like the Father did. She never drank alcohol, and she went to work. She did all she could to keep us together. I believe my saving grace was the work ethic I was taught by her.

My grandmother was fourteen years old when she gave birth to my mother. Subsequently, she had no role model. My mom was the first; seven more followed. My grandmother left the family when my mother was eighteen years old. She left eight children; the youngest was only one year old. By then my grandmother was thirty-two years old. She left with another man.

Today, I am very close to my mom. She is eighty-three years old. We are best friends, and I am grateful to still have her in my life.

Blessings

But I have also been blessed with gainful employment in my adult life. I have not lacked for any of the basic necessities. I have traveled on business, so I have seen much of our beautiful country. In spite of the abuses I have put my body through, miraculously I am relatively healthy. There is much more, but as a whole, *I am blessed*.

Over the years I have identified myself as a high-functioning dysfunctional. I don't want that label anymore.

I am on a mission to have a healthy, balanced relationship with the drug. My behavior so far has been submissive and weak. I have not had a strategy to win the battle and ultimately win the war. Well, I have outlined a plan now. I have no excuses going forward. It is time to put on the armor and fight the wars of addiction. This time, it is the drug war;

my own personal war on drugs.

I must remember that I am in control. I will use my brain and my heart as weapons of war to beat down the cravings and fight the urge to gorge and devour the drug. From now on, I dictate what happens in my life surrounding the drug. Does the drug win, or do I win?

I want to win!

In Closing

I have made gallons of lemonade in my lifetime …

I have insisted (to Jackie) over the years that I am not a product of my childhood. (The Queen of Denial speaks.) Truth is, I do have many traces of my childhood in my personality. Yes, I did break away from poverty and ignorance. And at least outwardly, I made a conscious effort to mainstream. Inside of me is the Little One who doesn't want to be deprived anymore, who doesn't want to be shoeless or hungry anymore, who is very present and overpowers me a lot. Additionally, she is still desperate to wear the coat of armor (the fat) to feel protected. She is at the source of my drug addiction. I must teach her to trust me. This can only come from my actions, not just my words.

I must always focus on the fact that I am not normal where food is concerned. I don't eat like normal people do. I struggle with every aspect of the food addiction. The biggest challenge I see is PORTION CONTROL. Because even though I may be eating the "right" foods, if I eat too much of (even) the right foods, I am defeating myself. Of course SUGAR is the main nemesis but the food drug in general is where this war lies. I want to win the battle I fight when I sit down to breakfast and lunch and dinner. Winning these small battles brings me closer to winning the war. Making right choices; I liken this to using the right weapons when I am on the battlefield. I will plan strategies in advance of stepping onto the battlefield.

Lists

I am a very visual person. I will hold myself accountable by preparing lists of the foods I want to consume during my program, the foods I will not allow in my body during my program, and things I want to accomplish during my program. I have chosen not to put my dreams on hold (deprivation) while I live in my program. I will pursue my goals as always. In other words, I want to live and produce as much as I want to day by day. There will not be any talk about putting off until tomorrow in relation to anything I want to accomplish. Life is happening today!

Edible Edibles List

- ❖ Vegetables

- ❖ Fruits

- ❖ Protein (fish, chicken, beef)

- ❖ Dairy (string cheese, nonfat milk, cottage cheese, etc.)

- ❖ Eggs (egg substitutes)

- ❖ Low-fat Frozen Meals (350 calories max)

- ❖ Low-fat Dessert (on Saturdays only)

This is a snapshot list only. There are many variables inside each bullet. Luckily, I like everything on this list and will incorporate satisfying meals from every food group. Being aware and prepared will help me to succeed. No more random stops at the supermarket, donut shop, or convenience store. The buck stops here. I will hold myself accountable, everyday.

Food For Thought

Have a king's breakfast, a queen's lunch, and a pauper's dinner.

Poison Dart List

Stop!

- ❖ Chocolate

- ❖ Pastries

- ❖ Fried Foods

- ❖ Candy

- ❖ Bread

- ❖ Pasta

- ❖ Fast Foods

- ❖ Pineapple and Watermelon (temporary)

My Goals

❖ I want to right-size and stay right-sized for the remainder of my life.

❖ I want to launch a new career.

❖ I want to continue to write. This is playtime for me!

❖ I want to take piano lessons.

❖ I want to travel to Germany, Ireland, France, and Spain.

❖ I want to continue to work until my mind and body cannot work anymore. I don't want to allow age to be a factor at all. Work has always been the center of my world. I admit it is another four-letter word, but it gives me fulfillment and a sense of accomplishment and meaning.

❖ I want to live life to its fullest and not say "what if" or "if only" when it comes time to close my eyes forever.

As we make our way in life, many of us will stop to ponder our experiences and we will ask the questions that challenge us and help us grow and mature. I want to acknowledge my weaknesses, applaud my strengths and rejoice in my successes. Most of all, always, always forgive myself when I stumble.

www.ingramcontent.com/pod-product-compliance
Lightning Source LLC
Chambersburg PA
CBHW020305290526
45784CB00003B/1366